SIRTFOOD Slim: Ignite Your Metabolism, Boost Energy, and Lose Weight Deliciously!

Unlock the Power of SIRT Foods and Transform Your Body with Mouthwatering Recipes and Expert Guidance

By

Emily Roberts

© **Copyright 2023 by (Emily Roberts) - All rights reserved.**

This document is geared towards providing exact and reliable information in regards to the topic and issue covered. The publication is sold with the idea that the publisher is not required to render accounting, officially permitted, or otherwise, qualified services. If advice is necessary, legal or professional, a practiced individual in the profession should be ordered.

- From a Declaration of Principles which was accepted and approved equally by a Committee of the American Bar Association and a Committee of Publishers and Associations.

In no way is it legal to reproduce, duplicate, or transmit any part of this document in either electronic means or in printed format. Recording of this publication is strictly prohibited and any storage of this document is not allowed unless with written permission from the publisher. All rights reserved.

The information provided herein is stated to be truthful and consistent, in that any liability, in terms of inattention or otherwise, by any usage or abuse of any policies, processes, or directions contained within is the solitary and utter responsibility of the recipient reader. Under no circumstances will any legal responsibility or blame be held against the publisher for any reparation, damages, or monetary loss due to the information herein, either directly or indirectly.

Respective authors own all copyrights not held by the publisher.

The information herein is offered for informational purposes solely, and is universal as so. The presentation of the information is without contract or any type of guarantee assurance.

The trademarks that are used are without any consent, and the publication of the trademark is without permission or backing by the trademark owner. All trademarks and brands within this book are for clarifying purposes only and are owned by the owners themselves, not affiliated with this document.

Table of Contents

Introduction 1

Chapter 1: Sirtfood Diet for Weight Loss and Increased Productivity 4

- 1.1 Reasons Why the Sirtfood Diet Works (According to Science) 4
- 1.2 How The Diet Helps to Lose Weight? 7
- 1.3 Achieving Mental Clarity and Better Brain Performance 8
- 1.4 Wide Range of Additional Health Benefits 10

Chapter 2: Understanding the Basics of Sirtfood Diet 13

- 2.1 What is a Sirtfood Diet? 13
- 2.2 The Origins and History of Sirtfood Diet 17
- 2.3 Is Sirtfood Diet Safe and Does It Live Up to its Hype? 28
- 2.4 Sirtfood Diet- A Diet Superior to Other Diets on the Market 33
- 2.5 Common FAQs about the Sirtfood Diet 50

Chapter 3: Getting Started with the Sirtfood Diet 52

- 3.1 Phases of Sirtfood Diet 54
- 3.2 Shopping List of Sirtfood Diet Foods 56
- 3.3 Sirtfood Diet – 1 week of food plan 61

Chapter 4: Delicious Sirtfood Diet Recipes 63

- 4.1 Breakfast Recipes 63
- 4.2 Sirtfood Diet Juices and Drinks 70
- 4.3 Lunch Recipes 71
- 4.4 Sirtfood Diet Salad Recipes 79
- 4.5 Dinner Recipes 84

- ❖ 4.6 SIRTFOOD DIET DESSERT RECIPES 92

Conclusion 95

Introduction

In a fast-paced world like ours, a world in which our lives are constantly getting busier and busier, individuals are constantly leaning towards the type of food that they can get access to very easily, e.g., fast food. But here lies the major problem, even though this food is very easily available almost all throughout the world, it is causing people to get obese. A disease to which major health hazards can find their roots in. This food, even though it is very tasty and accessible, packs in it a significant amount of calories, which don't even make the hunger die; this is a major problem. As a result of this, the individual consuming such a diet constantly finds himself in a state of hunger and constantly looks for similar sources of food to curb his hunger, which results in him over-consuming food. If you ever wanted to break such a cycle of consuming food over food without feeling any satisfaction or fulfillment and constantly seeing your body getting out of shape and degrade, then this book is definitely for you.

This book packs in it all the advice to combat weight gain through a fulfilling diet. This guide will help you get you in shape; it will also make your mental state clearer, and your self-esteem increased.

In this book, we will discuss a very popular and mainstream diet (Sirtfood) diet that definitely helps you lose weight as it has helped millions of other people lose weight, including celebrities such as the famous weight loss of sensational pop singer Adele.

What this revolutionary diet does is that it activates very special proteins inside the body called Sirtuins. These advanced proteins have the primary objective of saving body cells from dying under stress and are thought to regulate the aging process, inflammation, and metabolism. Sirtuins are considered to enhance the body's fat-burning, and boost metabolism actually results in a weight loss of seven pounds a week while retaining the muscle.

The Sirtfood diet was developed as "the alternative of traditional eating," as per Goggins. He and his wife, Glen Matten, were both "eating detractors" owing to their scientific background as medical scientists. The Sirtfood concept is based on triggering sirtuin genes rather than concentrating on weight loss. Sirtuins are proteins that belong to a class of enzymes. They trigger and are typically used to respond to stress and metabolism, a nutrition expert Kristin Kirkpatrick stated.

"The weight reduction is not the main objective, but as a part of the evolutionary rejuvenation of our cellular health, which ultimately restarts our metabolism," Goggins said. "Secondly, unlike other common diets where the emphasis is on taking food out, with Sirtfoods, we can only take advantage by feeding, and that ensures indulging in your delicious meals, not limiting them."

So, through the first chapters of the book, you will learn all about the Sirtfood diet and how it works, and as we move to forward chapters, you will learn how you could apply this diet for your benefit.

This book is also packed with tasty, delicious recipes for you to try and enjoy your Sirtfood diet journey.

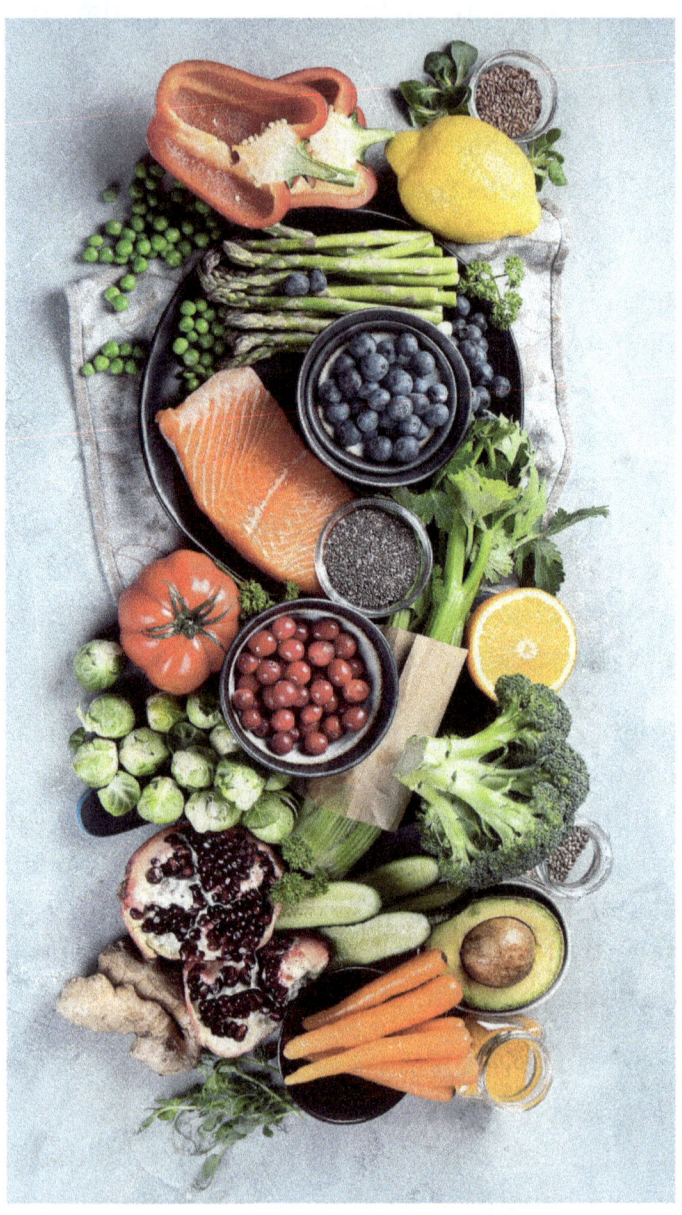

Chapter 1: Sirtfood Diet for Weight Loss and Increased Productivity

❖ 1.1 Reasons Why the Sirtfood Diet Works (According to Science)

In the health and wellness system, unique fad diets make loops. While some diets restrict food groups or nutrients strongly, others focus on the general well-being of the body. The sirt diet is one that has drawn the attention of many celebrities that personally endorse and profess the effects of certain diets. Adele has shocked us with her remarkable loss of weight. The singer was pictured in her slimmer avatar while on vacation with Harry Styles and James Corden on Anguilla's Caribbean Island. A source from The Sun indicates Adele is an immense fan of Sirtfood 's diet, which has played a major role in its dramatic weight loss. The sirt food diet may be a perfect choice for those who want to go on a safe path. That's what a sirt diet is.

The sirt food diet is based on research on SIRT or sirtuin. Research by the Glenn Laboratory for Aging Science in Massachusetts reveals the seven proteins found in the human body that regulate functions such as metabolism, inflammation, and lifespan. These proteins are found in the human body. The sirt food diet works on the assumption that certain plant compounds can increase these proteins. Such plants are referred to as Sirt foods. A combination of sirt foods and calorie restriction can lead to higher levels of sirtuin in your body, resulting in a quick loss of weight while maintaining muscle mass. According to the authors of sirtfood, Aidan Goggins and Glen Matten, "the diets of the slimmest, healthy, and longest-lived populations in the world – known as the blue zones – have previously shown that they have one thing in common, which they regard as their polyphenol content, is that they always have great richness in these precious plant nutrients." According to the authors, the effects of fasting and exercises can be replicated by activating a sirtuin (a.k.a 'skinny' gene) that contributes to the creation of the sirt diet.

Sirtfood Discovery

A study by the Institute of Human Nutrition and Food Science at Christian Albrecht's University, Kiel, Germany, showed a good dietary strategy for the prevention of chronic disease, combining Asian and Mediterranean sirt foods.

According to the authors, this will ensure the well-being and stable aging. Massachusetts, a collaborative study carried out by the Institute of Health Sciences, Shanghai, and the Glenn Laboratory for Aging Science, also found that sirtuin proteins increase the body's energy fat and improve insulin sensitivity.

How can you eat sirt food at home?

About 20 different foods can be classified as sirt foods. They include kale, red wine, strawberries, salt, soy, parsley, matcha green tea, buckwheat, turmeric, walnuts, coffee, etc. The Sirt food diet is followed in two stages. The first process involves seven days and requires a reduction in calories and high consumption of juice. It will lead to a weight loss beginning to jump, that will help us lose approximately 3.2 kg. During the first three days of this process, calorie intake should be limited to 1000 calories. Step two of the diet takes two weeks to eat three full meals of sirt meals and one green juice a day to proceed with the weight loss plan.

What if you eat a diet that is especially rich in sirt foods?

When it was discovered that a small group could replicate the effects of quickness and exercise by activating sirtuin in their bodies, the writers Aidan Goggin's and Glen Matten tested it and found that the participants lost an average of 3,18 kilograms in seven days while maintaining or even raising their mass muscles.

Production of sirtfood

Sirt foods include foods that are good for the human body, such as dark chocolate, green tea, and turmeric. Research published in the Clinical Hypertension Journal found that a high content of cacao can reduce the chance of heart disease and contribute to the fight against inflammation. A study published in Molecules found that turmeric is anti-inflammatory and can protect against chronic inflammatory diseases. We suggest that you consult a licensed nutritionist before you start on the fading diet band car since each body shape is unique and dietary requirements are different.

❖ 1.2 How The Diet Helps to Lose Weight?

Why eat sirtfood?

Although the diet is often hailed as easy to follow, because it contains red wine and dark chocolate, the guidelines are quite strict.

The sirt food plan relies on diets to reduce their calorie consumption and consume a certain list of foods to improve their metabolism. The three-week schedule involves an initial seven-day period and the two-week maintenance process, AKA. One of the most important elements is a green juice called by the founders "rocket fuel," which dietary followers have to make up to three times a day.

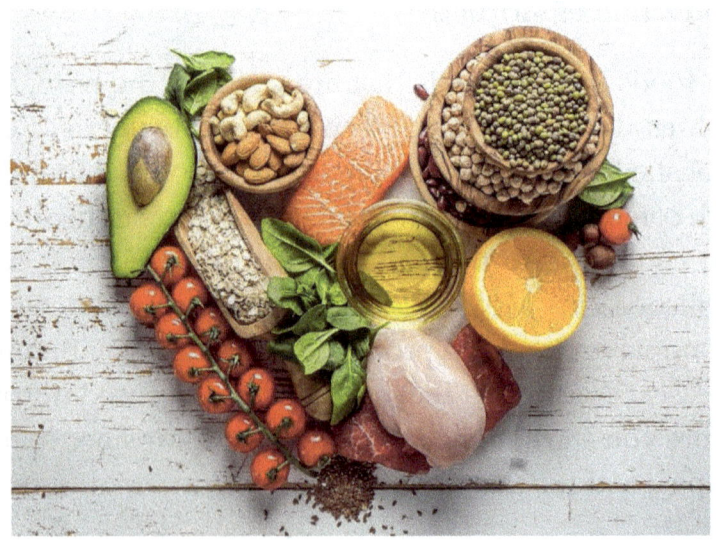

❖ 1.3 Achieving Mental Clarity and Better Brain Performance

It is known as the Sirtfood Diet and is rich in polyphenols that we enjoy from dark green vegetables and red fruits: buckwheat, tofu, green tea, dark chocolate, and red wine. These compounds activate genes known in our bodies as sirtuins that affect our lifespan. The longer we eat sirtfood, the more we live. It points out that the side effect of this is weight loss. There are several overlaps between the Sirtfood diet and the Mediterranean diet – the two are health-focused, but the Sirt diet is more precise and weighs away. Sirting (now a verb) focuses on savory green goods made of kale and matcha (among others) and a meal plan high in protein and vegetables, but low in carbs. The diet is not a weight loss diet but part of a three-week plan that aims to help us 'recover concentration, memory, and happiness.' The book is for the 'Scatterbrain' in the middle ages – that's me. It's good reading, though it's boring. The diet focuses on reducing meals and refined sugar as well as increasing the consumption of fruit and vegetables to 7 servings per day. The diet consists of a daily portion of oily fish to increase the intake of Omega 3. This reduces inflammation and improves brain function (I believe that's too much fish, but it's just for a short time). The food plan also suggests raising the intake of Omega 6: not all Omegas have been produced equal. Omega 6 increases swelling. Our ratio between Omega 6 and 3 should be about 2:1, but the ratio in the USA (the book is American) can be as high as 25:1. Omega 6s is found in processed oils and in manufacturing meat and milk, so the author recommends switching to organic eggs and meat or obtaining more proteins from plant sources. Other strategies to break up brain fog include minimizing the use of social media, meditation, community, friends, and family connections to the world and optimizing sleep.

RED WINE LENTILS (SERVES 4)

- One onion, finely chopped and peeled

- One carrot, skinned and thinly cut.

- One celery sticks, finely cut (optional)

- One garlic clove, peeled and thinly chopped

- Olive oil one tbs

- 250 g of puy lenses, rinsed

- 125ml red wine glass

- The stock of vegetables or water

- Small bunch of pink leaves, chopped

Sweat the first four ingredients in oil, and if they begin to stick, add a little water. Remove the lentils and add the red wine. Once absorbed, cover the lentils with stock or water and simmer until cooked, but with a small bite, adding more fluid if required. Remove the parsley and serve.

❖ 1.4 Wide Range of Additional Health Benefits

There is increasing evidence that sirtuin activators can have a wide variety of health benefits, build muscle, and suppress appetite. It improves memory, helps the body control blood sugar levels better, and removes damage from free radical molecules, which can build up in cells and result in cancer and other diseases. 'The beneficial effects of food and drink intake rich with sirtuin activators on decreasing the risk of chronic illness are substantially observational,' said Professor Frank Hu, a nutrition and epidemiology expert from Harvard University in a recent article in the journal Advances in Nutrition. A smart food diet is particularly appropriate as an anti-aging diet. Although there are sirtuin activators in the plant kingdom, there are only certain fruits and vegetables that have enough sirtfood. Sources include green tea, cacao powder, Indian peas, spinach, onions, and parsley. Many of the fruits and vegetables on display, such as tomatoes, avocados, bananas, lettuce, kiwis, carrots, and cucumbers in supermarkets, are actually quite low in sirtuin activators. However, this does not mean they are not worth eating as they bring several other benefits.

It's much more flexible to eat a diet packed with sirt foods than other diets. You can just eat a few sirt foods healthily. Or you could focus on them. Adding sirtfood could require more calories on low-calorie days with the 5:2 diet. One notable finding in a Sirt food diet study is that participants lost considerable weight without losing muscle. In reality, participants were always muscled, leading to a more developed and toned look. This is the beauty of sirts; fat burns are enabled, but also muscle development, maintenance, and repair are fostered. This contrasts entirely with other diets where weight loss is generally caused by fat as well as muscles, with the loss of muscles slowing down metabolism and making weight recovery more likely.

In the Sirtfood Diet, foods stimulating the SIRT1 genes are included. The diet is full of healthy foods that cause molecular weight loss and activate SIRT1 genes. This is how the diet of Sirtfood works:

1- Prevents fat accumulation: Adipokine expression is regulated by the SIRT1 genes. Fatty cells that affect insulin sensitivity and hunger and increase inflammation secrete Adipokines. Adipokine secretion is decreased by the SIRT1 gene activation by food in the Sirtfood diet. This prevents excessive accumulation of fat and premature starvation.

2- Mobilizes the fat: scientists have found that the foods included in the Sirtfood diet help morph the white adipose tissue stored in it into brown fat, which is easily mobilized and consumed as energy. The stored fat begins to melt and causes weight loss.

3- Excessive starvation regulates: Leptin is a hormone released from fat cells to signal a satiety brain. However, leptin resistance can sometimes inhibit this signal to the brain. This leads to constant famine and excessive consumption. Increased levels of SIRT1 in laboratory mice have been found to prevent age-related weight growth and to increase leptin sensitivity. Improving SIRT1 genes via

NAD+ intermediates (essential for activation of SIRT1) may help regulate excessive starvation by sensitizing the body to Leptin.

4- Improves insulin sensitivity: The cells' inability to react to insulin (the hormone that causes blood cell glucose to be absorbed) leads to increased blood sugar, obesity, and type 2 diabetes. Work shows that activating genes SIRT1 increases the sensitivity to insulin. In addition, this boosts metabolism, enhances the production of thyroid hormones, burns fatter, and protects against obesity caused by high-fat levels.

5- Reduces inflammation: Continuous inflammation can cause cells to function abnormally. This leads to fat build-up and co-morbidities associated with obesity (such as diabetes and heart disease). Enabled SIRT1 genes lead to inflammation reduction and to a reduction in the risk of heart disease and tumors.

Now that we are aware of how well the Sirtfood diet works, talk about the foods that help activate the genes SIRT1.

6- Lean muscle preservation: Activated SIRT1 genes can help maintain lean muscle mass while burning fat. Sirtuins (SIRT1 gene protein) increase the skeletal muscle mass. The SIRT1 genes activated promote muscle growth and recovery. Age-related muscle deterioration and muscle loss caused by exercise can also be avoided.

Chapter 2: Understanding the Basics of Sirtfood Diet

❖ 2.1 What is a Sirtfood Diet?

The Sirtfood diet, which was initially launched in 2016, remains a hot topic, involving followers adopting a diet rich in 'sirt foods.' Such unique foods function, according to the creators of the diet, by stimulating different proteins in the body, named sirtuins. Sirtuins are believed to protect the body's cells from dying while under stress, and are assumed to regulate inflammation, metabolic rate, and aging. Sirtuins are proposed to affect the body's fat burning and boost metabolism, leading in a weight loss of seven pounds a week while maintaining the muscle. However, some studies suggest this is unlikely to be merely a fat loss, but will bring change in skeletal muscle and liver glycogen stores instead.

Sirtfood Diet was created by two celebrity nutrition experts working with a fitness club in the United Kingdom. They promote the diet as a revolutionary new nutrition and fitness solution that works by turning on your "skinny gene." This concept is based on sirtuin research (SIRTs), a group of seven proteins found throughout the body that have been shown to regulate a multitude of roles including metabolism, inflammation and lifespan.

A pair of authors and nutrition specialists called Aidan Goggins and Glen Matten, who have always focused on eating a healthy diet rather than losing weight. The pair set out a meal plan in their new book The Sirtfood Diet which includes drinking three sirtfood green juices a day followed by healthy sirtfood-rich meals, such as a buckwheat and prawn stir-fry or smoked salmon sirt super salad.

The program claims consuming those foods would trigger your "skinny gene" course, and in 7 days you can lose 7 pounds. Foods such as kale, dark chocolate, and wine comprise a natural chemical called polyphenols which imitate the benefits of exercise and dieting. Strawberries, red onions, cinnamon and turmeric are potent sirt foods as well. The sirtuin route will activate these foods to help in losing weight. The science sounds enticing, but there is little research in reality to back up these claims. Plus, the expected weight loss pace in the first week is very high and not one or two pounds a week in accordance with the National Institute of Health 's recommendations on healthy weight loss.

Add healthy sirt foods to your diet for effective and sustained weight loss, amazing energy and healthy glow. Shift on the fat-burning abilities of your body, overload weight loss and help stave off the illness with this easy-to - follow diet created by dietary medicine specialists who have proved the influence of sirt foods. Dark chocolate, coffee, kale – all these are foods that activate sirtuins and turn on the body's so-called 'skinny gene' pathways. The Sirtfood Diet provides you with a simple, healthy way to eat for weight loss, delicious easy-to-make recettes and a long-term success review process. The Sirtfood Diet is a non-exclusion inclusion diet and sirtfoods are commonly affordable and available. This is a diet that empowers you to pick up your fork and knife and eat great nutritious food while seeing the advantages of health and weight loss.

There is mounting evidence that sirtuin modulators can have a wide variety of health advantages as well as building muscle and appetite suppression. This includes enhancing memory, helping the body to regulate blood glucose levels and cleaning up the harm done by free radical molecules that can grow in cells and contribute to cancer and other conditions.

'Substantial observation - based evidence exists for the positive effects of sirtuin-rich foods and beverages intake in reducing risk factors for chronic disease,' said Professor Frank Hu, a Harvard University consultant on nutrition and epidemiology, in a recent article in the journal Advances in Nutrition. A sirtfood diet is especially suited as an anti-aging regime. While activators of sirtuin are present in the plant kingdom, only some vegetables and fruits have sufficient amounts to qualify as sirt foods. Examples are including green tea, cocoa powder, turmeric for the Indian spice, kale, onions, and parsley. Many of the vegetables and fruits on display in grocery stores, such as tomatoes, avocados, bananas, lettuce, kiwis, carrots, and cucumber, are definitely rather low in modulators of sirtuin. However, this doesn't mean they aren't particularly tasty because they provide loads and loads of other advantages.

The benefit of consuming a sirtfood balanced diet is that it's much more versatile than other diets. Simply putting any sirtfoods on top you might eat well. Or you may be focused on getting them. The diet could require more calories on low calorie days, adding sirtfoods to claim.

Yet another remarkable finding from a sirtfood diet trial is that participants lost major body fat without having to lose muscle. In fact, gaining muscle definitely was common for participants, contributing to a more structured and toned look. That is sirtfoods' beauty; they stimulate fat burning, but they also encourage muscle growth, maintenance, and repair. This is in marked contradiction to other diets where weight loss usually comes from both muscle and fat, with muscle loss slowing down the metabolism and increasing the chance to regain weight.

❖ 2.2 The Origins and History of Sirtfood Diet

According to Goggins, the Sirtfood restaurant was founded as "the remedy to conventional diet." Due to their history as nutritious medical scientists, he and his spouse, Glen Matten, were both "diet sceptics." The Sirtfood diet is focused instead of relying on weight loss, on stimulating sirtuin genes. Sirtuins are proteins which belong to a family of enzymes. They activate and are typically used for stress and metabolism response, Kristin Kirkpatrick, a registered dietitian, explained.

"The weight loss is not the primary goal, but as a result of the genetic rejuvenation of our cellular wellness, which essentially resets our metabolism," Goggins said. "Secondly, unlike other popular diets where the focus is on cutting foods out, with Sirtfoods we can only reap the benefits by eating, and that means indulging in your favorite foods, not restricting them." Kirkpatrick, who works with the Cleveland Clinic in Ohio, said she had several patients who asked her about the Sirtfood diet. "The whole theory behind the diet is that some foods will activate these sirtuins which are related to the body's proteins." Kirkpatrick noted that the Sirtfood diet functions close to intermittent fasting diets, which have been shown to assist with weight loss, too.

Goggins said they became "increasingly concerned" about "increasingly extreme diet trends" and the foods that people "villainized" when he and Matten worked in a high-end private health club in London. "You'd have a fear of eating," he said. "And much of this has been about rising calorie consumption." They decided to make sure that people would be able to consume any of their favorite items while also having essential nutrients while developing the plan. "It is important that we not only get plenty of these foods in our diet but also ensure that our meals contain a variety of them as they are the synergy of their combination in meals and juices from which the real benefits come," said Googins.

The Sirtfood diet's true purpose is to load up one's meals with as many "sirtuin-activating nutrients" as possible. Sirtuin genes have been triggered in laboratory environments, but Kirkpatrick noted that although a pilot study by Goggins and Matten which studied 40 people on the diet, no other studies have been performed in humans. "Sirtfoods are all readily available, and plant foods accessible," Goggins said. "Some of the best Sirtfoods contain arugula, kale and parsley, almonds, walnuts, olive oil extra virgin, dark chocolate, curry seasoning, green tea, red wine and coffee."

Goggins and Matten recommend that you try to "sirtify" meals where possible and add Sirtfoods to favorite meals or replace regular ingredients with an alternative to Sirtfood. Kirkpatrick praised the food choices recommended in the diet. There are two phases to the diet. One should drink "three green Sirtfood juices and one full meal rich in Sirtfoods" daily for the first three days on the diet, for a total of just 1,000 calories per day.

People should enhance their intake to 1,500 calories a day on days four through seven by consuming "two green juices and two meals." According to Goggins, during this phase, people lose 7 pounds in seven days, although Kirkpatrick noted that anyone eating just 1,000 calories a day would see weight-loss effects regardless of what they consumed.

The actual food is good," Kirkpatrick said. "The first phase depends heavily on green juices and 'no more than 1,000 calories'. Anything with 1,000 calories and pretty severe caloric limitation will result in weight loss, but the body will bounce back. The quest for alternate fuels on the body. You're more likely to gain weight once you get into those later phases and start relaxing the motivation you've had in weeks one and two.' Goggins said, though, that once the phases are over, the diet focuses more on what you eat, rather than how much. "While the initial one-week phase has a calorie restriction, there's no maintenance count," he said. "We 're eating now as we've always been meant to, and we've been eating throughout history."

As experts in nutritional medicine and pharmacy, Aidan and Glen have long been fascinated by the natural compounds found in plant foods, known as polyphenols, and how they can be harnessed to improve health and even treat disease. They were particularly fascinated by how plants and polyphenols were being vigorously exploited by the drug industry to create new drugs for their medicinal properties, yet they ha Intriguingly, the diets of the slimmest, healthiest, and longest-lived populations around the world – known as the Blue Zones – had previously shown that the one thing they had in common was that they were always very rich in these precious plant nutrients, about five times the intakes we consume in the West.

Aidan and Glen described the foods with the highest amounts of such potent polyphenols triggering sirtuins and referred to this freshly found category of wonder foods as 'Sirtfoods,' and posed the question: what will be the effects if you eat a diet exclusively abundant in all these products? When they first studied this, they were surprised at the findings. That was of course well and fine for short-term performance, so what about long-term outcomes? The findings from one of the highest and greatest dietary experiments ever performed were published at the same period, and they were stunning. The research found that the risk of heart disease, diabetes, obesity and early death slashed dramatically following a Sirtfood-rich Mediterranean diet. The findings were greater than any prior dietary research reported, and much preferable to any medications that might yield any test. That was the last piece Aidan and Glen had been looking for at the jigsaw. They set out to share their method with the world with that in place, and so the Sirtfood Diet was born.

But that was only the beginning of a Sirtfood tale. The actual consequences in life became evident when hundreds, then thousands, and tens of thousands of people adopted the plan. Diet participants witnessed fast and persistent weight loss. But they also had life-changing health benefits, recovery of their ailments, and major changes of their well-being, more than that. Word has since spread far and wide, seeing the Sirtfood Diet becoming an international bestseller, and changing the way the world eats, one delicious mouthful at a time.

Whether you're trying to lose weight or becoming more conscious about feeding your body, knowing Sirtfoods is crucial. Sirtfoods are a group of nutrient-rich foods that help regulate your metabolism, burn fat and muscle gain. THE SIRTFOOD DIET writers Aidan Goggins and Glen Matten share what you need to know about Sirtfoods.

When we cut back on calories, this causes an energy shortage that stimulates what is known as the "skinny gene," causing a torrent of positive change. It places the body in a kind of survival state where fat is prevented from being processed and regular development cycles are placed on hold. Instead, the body is turning its attention to burning up its fat stores and switching on powerful housekeeping genes that repair and rejuvenate our cells, effectively giving them a spring clean. The upshot is weight loss and heightened disease resistance. But cutting calories, as many dieters know, comes at a cost. Reducing energy intake in the short term is causing hunger, irritability, fatigue, and muscle loss. Long-term restriction on calories is causing our metabolism to stagnate. This is the collapse of all calorie-restrictive diets and paves the way for a piling back on the weight. For these reasons, 99 percent of dietitians are doomed to long-term failure. All of this has led us to ask a major question: is it possible to trigger our slim genes with all the wonderful benefits they bring and all those disadvantages without having to adhere to an extreme calorie restriction?

Enter Sirtfoods, a group of wonder-foods newly discovered. Sirtfoods are especially rich in special nutrients that can activate the same skinny genes in our bodies when we consume them as calorie restriction does. Those genes are called sirtuins. They first came to light in a landmark study in 2003 when researchers discovered that resveratrol, a compound found in red grape skin and red wine, dramatically increased the yeast 's life span.2 Incredibly, resveratrol had the same effect on longevity as calorie restriction, but this was achieved without reducing energy intake. Studies have since indicated that resveratrol can be extended. Early-stage experiments indicate that resveratrol defends against the harmful consequences of high-calorie, high-fat and high-sugar diets; encourages safe aging by preventing age-related diseases; and improves mobility. Essentially, the effects of calorie restriction and exercise have been proved to be mimicked.

Red wine was dubbed as the first Sirtfood with its rich resveratrol material, describing the health benefits associated with its intake, and even why people who drink red wine get less weight. This is only the beginning of the Sirtfood tale, though. The field of health science was at the cusp of something major with the detection of resveratrol and the pharmaceutical industry lost little time getting on board. Researchers have started screening thousands of different chemicals for their capacity to activate our sirtuin genes. That revealed a number of natural plant compounds with significant sirtuin-activating properties, not just resveratrol. It was also found that a given food could contain a whole spectrum of these plant compounds, which could work together to both aid absorption and maximize the sirtuin-activating effect of that food. This had been one of the big resveratrol mysteries. Resveratrol experimenting scientists often needed to use far higher doses than we know when consumed as part of the red wine to provide a benefit. Nevertheless, as well as resveratrol, red wine contains a range of other natural plant compounds including high amounts of piceatannol as well as quercetin, myricetin and epicatechin, each of which has been shown to activate our sirtuin genes independently and, more importantly, to work in coordination.

The dilemma for the pharmaceutical companies is that they cannot sell the next major breakthrough product as a collection of nutrients or foods. So instead they invested hundreds of millions of dollars in the hopes of uncovering a Shangri-La pill to develop and conduct tests of synthetic compounds. Multiple studies of sirtuin-activating drugs for a multitude of chronic diseases are currently underway, as well as the first-ever FDA-approved trial to investigate whether a medicine can slow aging. If history has taught us anything, it's that we shouldn't hold much hope for this pharmaceutical ambrosia, as tantalizing as that may seem. The nutrition and wellness companies have continuously sought to imitate the effects of foods and diets by separated nutrients and medications. And it has come up short again and again. Why wait ten more years for these so-called wonder drugs to be licensed, and the inevitable side effects they bring, when right now we have all the incredible benefits available through the food we eat at our fingertips? So while the pharmaceutical industry is pursuing a drug-like magic bullet relentlessly, we need to retrain our focus on dieting.

Participants in our Sirtfood Diet trial lost an impressive 7 pounds over the initial 7 days including muscle and muscle function increases. This dramatic effect on fat-burning, while promoting muscle, is one of the reasons why our Sirtfood diet has become so popular with anyone who wants to get lean and in great shape, just as the elite athletes and models who have championed this way of eating have. In addition to fat burning, Sirtfoods often has the remarkable potential to satiate hunger naturally, rendering it the ideal option for a healthier weight and long-term sustainability. But just thinking about it as a diet for weight loss is missing the point. That is a lifestyle that is as well-being-related as waistlines. The good 'side effects' from this form of eating are improved stamina, smoother skin, feeling more alert, and better sleep. Sometimes the benefits are even more notable, including cases where metabolic diseases have been reversed in the longer term following the diet. These are their health-enhancing effects that studies show them to be more powerful than prescription drugs in chronic disease prevention, with advantages in diabetes, heart disease, and Alzhemier's, to name just a few. It's no wonder that it's well-established that the cultures that eat the most Sirtfoods in the world are the leanest and healthiest.

The bottom line is clear: If you want to make the body more efficient, leaner and safer, and build the groundwork for good fitness and disease tolerance, then the Sirtfood Diet is for you.

Goggins and Matten find in their own studies that participants quickly lose weight following a high-sirt food diet (admittedly it is calorie-restricted within the first week).

More importantly, without increasing their exercise, they gained muscle mass and showed lower blood sugars and blood fats. They also reported having more energy, sleeping better, looking better, and having no hunger problems. Goggins and Matten soon realized that these sirt foods are present in the kitchens of those communities that claim the lowest incidence of obesity and disease in the world, most clearly in the Mediterranean diet. It is worth noting that these foods are not unusual or inaccessible for the most part, and the eating plan is simple and reasonable enough to fit in with any other food you might follow – 5:2, low carb, Paleo, vegetarian, even vegan or gluten-free.

If you choose to strictly follow that diet, you'll need a juicer. You'll drink the green juice three times a day for the first three days, with one meal. Days 4 to 7 call for two beverages and two meals so you can add only one juice to your usual three meals afterwards. Apparently weight loss of half a stone in the first week is likely, and that includes putting on an average of two pounds of muscle. Exercise shouldn't be strenuous, though Goggins and Matten suggest that everyone prepare for general good health in half an hour a day. The only other suggestion is to try to stop eating by 7 pm, as calories are processed less efficiently by the body as the day goes on. And, while sirtfoods are plant foods, they also point out that you need to combine them with some form of protein to get maximum benefits from both. We all know that processed meat should be avoided, and red meat should be kept once or twice a week, but poultry, eggs (and milk in moderation) are fine, as are lentils and soy, beans and nuts of course. Sirtfoods also have a particularly beneficial omega-3 oils relationship, so include oily fish two to three times a week.

Although I'm concerned with specific plant foods and weight management, a fascinating and large-scale recent research found that those eating the most flavonoids were the most likely to sustain their weight or even lose weight as they reached middle age, so only a handful of berries a day, say, is enough to have some impact.

Flavonoids are a category of antioxidant plant chemicals contained especially in bananas, blackcurrants, oranges, citrus fruits, dark chocolate, beans, tomatoes, tea and red wine – all substantially sirt foods – as well as radishes, prunes, grapes and rhubarb. Researchers conclude that flavonoids may have a positive impact on intestinal bacteria, and is evolving as the main story of metabolism and weight management – more over the next several weeks.

Top rated sirtfoods

Kale, celery, parsley, rocket, red chicory, lovage, red onions, bird's eye chillies, capers, turmeric (mix with black pepper and some type of nutrient-activating oil), olives, soy, quinoa, extra virgin olive oil, walnuts, buckwheat, (and all nuts), blackcurrants, (and strawberries and all berries), citrus fruit, apples, green tea, and in moderation red wine, coffee and cocoa.

Ideas for Recipe (to serve one)

Green Juice

Juice 2 of kale with a few of rocket, small amount parsley and lavage, 3 celery stalks and seeds, and half a green apple. Add 1/2 lemon juice, and 1/2 tsp of green tea matcha powder.

Sirt Muesli

Mix 20 g buckwheat flakes with 10 g buckwheat puffs (health food shop), 15 g of desiccated coconut, 15 g of chopped walnuts, 40 g of chopped dates, 10 g of cocoa, 100 g of chopped strawberries and 100 g of greek yogurt or soya yogurt).

Mix 100 g of smoked salmon with minced celery, celery leaves or lavage, red onion, half an avocado, parsley, capers and walnuts, olive oil and lemon juice, then serve on rocket then chicory leaves.

Stir Fry Prawn

Cook 150 g in a little shelled prawns, olive oil and soya sauce, and put them aside. Cook 75 g of soba (buckwheat) noodles as specified, in boiling water. Meanwhile, in a little bit more fry chopped garlic, bird's eye chili, olive oil (be very careful with these, they 're hot), red onion, celery, ginger, kale, and green beans and add 100ml of stock. Bring to the boil, simmer with prawns and noodles for a minute or two.

❖ 2.3 Is Sirtfood Diet Safe and Does It Live Up to its Hype?

Yes, Sirtfood is not only safe, it has a vast array of health benefits including cancer fighting, as we know it activates sirtuins that are specialized proteins and have a wide range of health benefits for human bodies. Sirtuins are stress-responsive proteins that control various post-translational modifications (PTMs) and are therefore called master regulators of several cellular processes, according to the research done. They are considered to extend lifespan as well as control the growth of random tumours. As both aging and cancer are linked with altered stem cell function, it is worth investigating the possibility of sirtuin participation in these incidents being influenced by their functions in stem cells. Research to date suggests that individual members of the sirtuin family can regulate embryonic, hematopoietic and other adult stem cells differently in a context specific to the tissue and cell type. Sirtuin-driven modulation of both the cell differentiation and signaling pathways previously involved in stem cell maintenance was identified where the biological outcome was decided by the downstream effectors involved. Similarly, diverse roles in cancer stem cells (CSCs) were reported, depending on the original tissue. This analysis illustrates existing awareness that positions sirtuins at stem cell intersection, ageing and cancer. By outlining the abundance of stem cell-related roles for individual sirtuins in different contexts, our purpose was to provide an indication of their significance in relation to cancer and aging, and to generate a clearer picture of their therapeutic potential. Lastly, we propose future directions that will contribute to a better understanding of sirtuins and thus further unravel the full repertoire of sirtuin functions in both normal stem cells and CSCs.

Sirtuins and stem cells

Embryonic stem cells and development

Histone acetylation undergoes dynamic changes during embryonic stem cell differentiation (ESCs), and as a result appears to play a significant role in development. In particular, ESCs exhibit higher histone acetylation levels than lineage-restricted and more differentiated cells (Efroni et al., 2008). It is not unexpected, therefore, that sirtuins were related with the production and differentiation of ESCs. It is important to note here that in most sirtuin-knockout mice, early embryonic development is reported to be normal; however, Sirt1 knockout results in significant lethality during or shortly after birth, with severe developmental deficiencies (Cheng et al., 2003; Haigis et al., 2006b; Mostoslavsky et al., 2006; Lombard et al., 2007; Vakhrusheva et al., 2008; Du et al., 2011; Kim et al., 2006). As a result, SIRT1 is considered in these processes to be the most important sirtuin, and is therefore the best studied in this context. Since Sirt1 is highly expressed in ESCs before being down-regulated during differentiation by miRNAs (Saunders et al., 2010), it is thought to play a role in preserving stemness of ESCs and appears to be involved in developmental programs after differentiation of ESCs (Table 1). The role of SIRT1 in ESC differentiation varies depending on environmental conditions – loss of Sirt1 does not induce differentiation under normal conditions; however, under oxidative stress, Sirt1 mediates the maintenance of stemness promoting mitochondrial over the nuclear translocation of p53 and maintaining the expression of Nanog (Han et al., 2008; Calvanese et al., 2010). SIRT1 is a known component of the Polycomb Repressive Complex 4 (PRC4), which suppresses developmental genes in ESCs (Kuzmichev et al., 2005) and also binds development-associated gene promoters in ESCs such as TBX3 and PAX6 where it contributes to gene silencing. The role of SIRT1 in the cell reprogramming of somatic cells to induced pluripotent stem cells (iPSCs) was also investigated as a result of its ability to regulate stemming and pluripotency factors. Both SIRT1 overexpression and treatment with the established sirtuin activator resveratrol have been shown to enhance iPSC generation performance, whereas Sirt1 knockdown exerts counteracting action. This effect is associated with p53 deacetylation and increased expression of the Nanog (Lee et al., 2012).

Provided that the equilibrium between cell differentiation and self-renewal is crucial to the preservation and tissue regeneration of adult stem cells, studies have revealed a role for sirtuins as differentiation regulators in many cell types. In normal neural stem cell differentiation (NSCs), SIRT1 translocates to the nucleus where it interacts with the corepressor nuclear receptor (N-CoR) to block Notch-Hes1 signaling and promote neuronal differentiation (Hisahara et al., 2008) (Table 1). However, tension factors in the stem cell differentiation pathways appear to have a specific impact on

SIRT1 functions, also within the same cell group. Thus, mild oxidation induces SIRT1 to bind to Hes1 and guides NSC segregation against the astroglial lineage rather than the neuronal lineage (Prozorovski et al., 2008), which may promote astrogliosis and healing in reaction to brain and spinal cord injury.

Emerging evidence suggests that sirtuins could be placed at stem, aging and cancer crossroads. This is based on the multiplicity of functions they regulate in both normal stem cells and CSCs. However, it is clear that we are just beginning to appreciate the importance of identifying specific processes in a tissue, cell type, and genetic-specific context that are regulated by the different members of the sirtuin family. This could be necessary to gain a better understanding of their role and to fill the current gaps in knowledge in the field. With that in mind, it is worth noting that most of the previous studies followed a targeted approach to elucidating sirtuin-regulated mechanisms. To do so, they focused on either unraveling how sirtuins regulate signaling pathways / processes that are already involved in stemness, or exploring whether well-established sirtuin functions play a significant role in stem cells. In this direction, it could be proposed that more mechanistic insights would be provided by implementing unbiased high-throughput experimental approaches.

In the past, proteomics was used to identify sirtuin-specific proteins and substrates which interact. During mitosis, SIRT2 's regulatory role on anaphase-promoting complex (APC / C) was identified based on a proteomics approach that revealed its interaction with complex proteins including the APC activator proteins Cdc20 and Cdh1 (Kim et al., 2011). Proteomics have recently been used to elucidate the interaction landscape of the mitochondrial sirtuin protein, showing that this experimental approach can uncover novel functions and/or substrates (Yang et al., 2016). Thus, similar approaches on stem and progenitor cells or CSCs could be suggested to identify novel sirtuin functions. In addition, recent advances in high-resolution proteomics based on mass spectrometry have enabled acetylome to be studied under various experimental conditions establishing acetylation as an equally widespread PTM as phosphorylation (Kim et al., 2006; Choudhary et al., 2009, 2014). Given that similar methods have allowed sirtuin-specific targets for deacetylation to be established (Hebert et al., 2013; Vassilopoulos et al., 2014), it would be logical to conclude that studying acetylome in the form of stem cells / progenitors or CSCs would uncover new functions / substrates controlled at the post-translation stage. Similarly, a thorough characterization of target genes epigenetically controlled by sirtuins in different subcellular populations may help form new directions in this area and supplement previous systematic research centered on studying the transcriptome, DNA methylome, and histone modifications in stem cells (Sun et al., 2014). These research can potentially include fresh perspectives into both aging and cancer.

❖ 2.4 Sirtfood Diet- A Diet Superior to Other Diets on the Market

Let's realize, how does the human body actually find that many distinct forms of slimming down?

Each year there appears to be some revolutionary diet rolling in hot off the press with the encouragement of several big celebrities. It makes its big debut, and thanks the front of every popular magazine in the checkout line of the grocery store. Another fitness advocate who featured on a well-known chat show discussing the evidence behind this modern form of dieting, as though it were a brand different discovery

Still, you can't help but wonder if perhaps this one is going to be the trick that will help you get back into your favorite pair of jeans from a long time before childbearing. Or your days of eating whatever you want the heck you want without earning a single pound are over, at least before adulthood says sorry honey.

There have been two eating programs over the past three years and have been fighting it out in the spotlight. There's a low-carb, high-fat Keto diet and a "skinny gene" diet that boosts SIRTfood.

What divides the two? What are the best plans for your wellbeing and weight loss? What makes a "skinny gene" in the world?

Let's discover everything there's to learn about every diet to address your questions. The following is your ultimate guide to all of the keto, sirt and the science behind it.

What is the Keto Diet?

Let's continue with the keto diet, or ketogenic diet. In short, a keto diet consists of low carbohydrate intake, moderate proteins, and high fat foods. True keto peeps strive to eat 20 g or less of carbohydrates a day-consuming most of their calories from healthy fat. Invented by Peter Huttenlocher back in the 1970s, the idea behind this is that your body will enter a "ketosis" state. What is it that now? It is yet another sophisticated way of suggesting that the body ceases depending on glycogen and starts to eat carbon instead. Basically, when you limit your intake of carb and calories, your body (especially your liver) produces tiny molecules called ketones that work when your blood sugar levels are low, to provide your body with energy.

Ketones are made from fat, so your body is reprogrammed to run on fat, as opposed to glucose on this diet. Through restricting your calorie consumption and, in a sense, teaching the body to use fat for food, it can then start consuming fat reserves in the body as it requires energy.

Sounds sensible, right? Now ... let's just switch gears and we will talk about SIRT!

What's the diet for sirtfood?

Before we learn about SIRT's diet plan, let us know that that diet encourages you to eat dark chocolate and red wine (in moderation). How can that be? This new diet, created by nutritionists Aidan Goggins and Glen Matten, involves a fair amount of "sirtfoods." In other words, foods that make the body make a protein called Sirtuin. These special small proteins help reduce inflammation and protect our cells against stress damage. Oh, so sirtuins to cells like we have red wine ... Everything's making sense! A Sirt food diet will significantly improve your metabolism and burn fat quickly. After this diet plan was started, men and women reportedly drop up to seven pounds per week. In contrast to the ketogenic diet, the diet for sirtfood is divided into two phases. During the first three days, you have to cut your daily intake to 1000 calories with three green sirtfood juices plus one sirtfood meal per day.

Day 4-7, when you enjoy two green juices and one sirt-food meal per day, you can increase your intake to 1500 calories. The next two weeks will then be referred to as the recovery period, and the body will begin to gradually lose weight. This process is called a 'skinny gene' when our body's usual source of energy runs low by reducing calories. However, there are few and many studies behind sirtfood. Job is needed to better understand Sirtuin 's effects on our well-being. Having said that, the sirt food diet creates big waves, and people around the world see results. Celebrities such as pop singer Adele, who lost almost 50 pounds to eat SIRT, show that this weight loss plan, along with the practice, actually works.

Keto Diet: What Can You Eat

And now the part you all waited for ... what you could eat! A keto diet includes a wide range of high-fat foods, which are probably already in the fridge.

- **Low carbon veggies**

Fun Eat your greens! Fun Eat your greens! Asparagus, Brussels, and broccoli are all nutrient-dense vegetables you can consume in the ketogenic diet in abundance. The list continues. It is a keto-friendly veggie as long as the carbohydrate count is low.

- **Seafood**

Salmon, shrimp, halibut ... all full of keto-friendly and vitamin-rich. Just look for some shellfish like palms, moules, octopus, and oysters, because the carbohydrates are high.

- **Attorneys**

This delicacy of California is a pleasure to enjoy on the keto diet. It is rich in fatty acids and omega 3. Nice as a snack or combined with some veggies or smoothie.

- **Cheese**

Ultimo, some of you, say Hallelujah! Yes, because of its high-fat content, the keto diet allows cheese. The best options are Mozzarella and cheddar cheeses. Beware of fried cheese and other high-sugar dairy foods.

- **Honeycomb**

The other great source of fat, omega-3 fatty acids, and important nutrients, eggs are an enjoyable breakfast or a midday snack.

- **Poultry and meat**

THE category is a staple of the ketogenic diet. They have no carbohydrates and are full of useful vitamins. Choose foods higher in fat, like ribeye steaks and chicken thighs.

- Greek Yogurt Simple

Anything else wonderful to enjoy, Greek Yoghurt. It's nearly a dessert. Treat yourself.

- **Cheese Cottage**

Not only a way to get fats but helps to lower inflammation and cure dull muscles after exercise.

- **Coconut oil Coconut oil**

If you didn't know, cocoa oil is a perfect substitute for other cooking oils because it is easier to burn at such high temperatures. You know, it's great to rub a sunburn when you bounce around on the beach, showing your new bikini body from a keto diet.

Sirtfood Diet: What should you eat?

enjoy following the Keto diet, let 's find out more about the mysterious "SIRTfood," so we can compare both diet plans.

- **Dates of Medjool**

Medjool dates are recommended in sirt foods, unlike other dates, as they are caramel-like in taste and texture. They have numerous health benefits and are a popular choice during the sirt food diet. They are great for smoothies or for snacks that satisfy your sweet tooth. They are also an excellent alternative tea or coffee sweetener.

- **Green Tea**

There is a key component of the Sirt food diet, green tea, consists of a significant bioactive sirtuin called catechin that reduces oxidative stress and increases metabolism. It acts as a suppressant of appetite and picks me up well. The better you drink!

- **Dark chocolate (must be 85% cocoa at least)**

Not rich in flavor and polyphenols – eat moderate amounts of dark chocolate on the sirt food diet with no concern. Make sure that the cocoa content is at least 85 percent or higher.

- **Tropical fruits**

We already know that citrus fruits are rich in vitamins, nutrients, and fiber, but now we are aware that they are very high in polyphenols, and that they are helpful in burning fat and becoming slender.

- **Apple**

Up to you know what they mean. You know what they say. An apple holds the doctor away one day, and an apple a day helps to prevent weight gain.

- **Parsley**

This herb is full of nutrients and antioxidants. It promotes bone safety and protects your vision. Use parsley for garnishing or combining it with other cooked vegetables to help your well-being.

- **Coal.**

As one of the world's most nutrient-dense foods, kale can be used on a diet of sirtfood abundantly. Enjoy it as a salad in a smoothie.

- **Turmeric**

It is a welcome addition to this dietary plan to a medicinal herb with anti-inflammatory effects. A dosage of 500 to 2,000 milligrams of turmeric a day is safe to eat.

- **Heavenly fruits**

Blueberries, the fruit of the planet, is a refreshing pleasure to enjoy this diet. They 're also great for hydration and vitamin-filled shock.

- **Red Wine**

Last but not least, red wine is welcomed on a Sirt food diet with open arms (in moderation, of course). This is not the only sirt food you can enjoy. Others include coffee, arugula, chilies, walnuts, and much more, but you get the spit!

- **Caps**

Up Bet you knew that capers were an unbelievably healthy superfood. They can be used to treat diabetes, fungal infections, arthritis, and other diseases.

Keto Diet Benefits vs. Sirtfood Diet Benefits

These two common diets tend to encourage you to take advantage of a wide variety of diets that other diets enable you to cut to meet your weight loss goals. They deliver a much more practical and satisfying menu than the diet for cold soup. The big question now is: which one would be better for you and your health? The keto diet helps you lose weight and has other safety advantages. It can help to improve acne, improve heart and brain function, and reduce your risk of life-threatening diseases such as certain cancers. It has also been said that it helps to reduce seizures in young children.

Studies have shown that you can stick with a mainly ketogenic eating plan for the longer term, but it is important to your overall health to add more carbohydrates, such as potatoes, fruits, and beans.

On the other hand, a diet of SIRTfood was also promoted to achieve a rapid loss of weight. It protects you from chronic diseases and has anti-aging skills. If you are strict with this diet or not, the addition of these rich nutrients in your diet will improve your health.

However, this diet is not realistic for a number of reasons over the long term. The super-low calorie and low carbon intakes can be unhealthy, and research to assess the impact it has on our bodies is still very necessary.

Ultra Keto Diet

The high-fat, low-carb Keto Diet overtook Google's trendiest diet searches last year. This year, the "Keto Super" diet, which includes vitamins, entered the ten most frequently searched diets. "The ketogenic diet of carbohydrates is rather small, and the body becomes very high in fat – fat becomes eaten rather than glucose for food.," said Wright. "Keto Diet has been shown to minimize heaviness as any diet that limits whole food groups will lead to lower caloric intakes as a result of a lower diet. A side effect of ketosis decreases appetite, thus contributing to lower weight." But the diet has risks. "With the absence of carbohydrate-containing foods like fruit, vegetables, whole grain and beans, ketogenic diets can lead to some vitamin- and mineral deficiencies and may adversely affect intestinal health," mentioned Wright. "There have also been reports of losing muscle mass for people who adopt a ketogenic diet, which is especially troubling for older adults."

Hunnes believes that a keto-based diet is not balanced. "I don't agree that this is a safe option since our primary energy source is evolutionarily dependent on glucose. A high-fat, high-protein diet is not at all beneficial for us. I do not suggest a ketogenic diet in the strongest possible words," she said. Both Wright and Hunnes note that children who have seizures and follow the diet according to their doctor's medical instructions are the only ones who may actually benefit from a keto-based diet. "The ketogenic diet has been shown to treat severe epilepsy in infants and children under medical supervision successfully," Wright said.

No Carbs, No Sugar

Singer Jennifer Lopez revealed earlier this year that she was attempting to fight no carbohydrates and no sugar for ten days. Lopez encouraged her followers to join her days into her diet. Experts claim, however, that some carbs are required. "Our brains, like our muscles, are dependent on glucose from carbohydrates for healthy functioning," said Hunnes. "This form of diet is not safe. Of course, it is safe to reduce or prevent sugar but not to restrict all carbohydrates." Wright agreed.

The problem for many is the type and amount of carbs consumed. Instead of simple sugars, like soda and candy, it is important to emphasize complex carbs, such as whole grains, rice, beans, vegetables, and fruits.

"Along with body fuel capacity, carbohydrates also provide vitamins, minerals, and fiber," added Wright. "Carbohydrates are important and must not be taken off the diet. Instead, pick healthy carbohydrates and monitor portions. Excessive carbohydrates will add extra calories and cause diabetic high blood sugars." Wright suggests that a suitable portion of carbohydrate is half a cup of pasta instead of a whole dish or one-third to two-thirds rice rather than a whole bowl.

Longevity and Sirtuins

Studies of, for example, mice, bees, and flies have shown that SIRT1 can have a significant health and longevity effect. And another recent study showed that SIRT3 levels increased when study participants fasted daily, i.e., decreased their calorie intake to just 500 per day for two days per week. However, the study was small, with only 24 participants, so more research is required to confirm these findings. "Research on how diverse foods can affect how our genes express themselves still takes place in their early childhood, and this is only a fragment," says Farah Cleret, a nutritionist. "A healthy diet never should be limited to how one gene is affected, as several different factors are also at stake. It is also important to keep the diet fresh and varied and to avoid refined and unhealthy foods when possible."

Resolutions of the Year

As 2020 is in the middle and this year goals and resolutions begin to be reached, all experts who have spoken to Healthline focus on bringing about sustainable lifestyle changes and not on extreme diets. "Do not make this an artificial time for you to start good customs, and be aware that the best diet you can have is the diet you can stay on for long periods," said Kirkpatrick. "Depart from the term diet and think of a change in lifestyle that will sustain continued success," said Wright. Look at something like the Mediterranean dietary plan, which includes planting with vegetables, fruit, whole grains, and lean fish and meats and uses healthy fats. Combined with exercise, this plan is a system in which you can live and achieve your health aims.

So how is this diet different from the Mediterranean diet?

Many people claim that the sirt diet is a combination of the Mediterranean diet (olive petroleum, plenty of fresh meat, fruit, and fish) and the Asian diet, i.e., a diet full of soy products such as tofu, green tea or oily fish. Some may also suggest that a Sirt food diet often needs to include some fasting, as other research has shown that fasting increases some sirtuins.

The truth is that a so-called Sirt food diet can alter any kind of diet that can increase the behavior of sirtuins. Research has also shown that this is olive oil, dark chocolate, leafy green vegetables, blueberries, citrus fruits, tofu, oily fish, and sometimes a red glass of tea.

Sirts are almost all healthy choices, and their antioxidant or anti-inflammatory properties can result in certain health benefits. However, eating just a few particularly healthy foods cannot meet every nutritional requirement of your body. The Sirtfood Diet is overly restrictive and does not have specific and special health benefits over any other diet.

In addition, it is typically not recommended to eat only 1000 calories without the supervision of a doctor. Even a daily diet of 1,500 calories is too restrictive for many. The diet requires up to three green juices a day as well. While juices can provide a good source of vitamins and minerals, they also contain virtually no healthy fibers like whole fruit and vegetables, as well as sugar. Moreover, sipping on juice all day long is a bad idea for your blood sugar and teeth. Not to mention that the diet is so limited in calories and food choice that the protein, vitamins, and minerals, particularly during the first phase, are more than likely deficient. This diet can be difficult to adhere to for the entire three weeks due to the low-calorie levels and limited food choices. In addition to the high initial cost of buying a juicer, the book, and some rare and expensive ingredients along with the time it takes to prepare certain foods and juices, this diet will become impossible for many.

SUMMARY: The Sirtfood Diet encourages healthy food but restricts calories and food choices. It also requires a lot of juice to be drunk, which is not a sound recommendation.

Advantages of Sirtfood Diet over Other Diets

During the initial seven days, participants in our Sirtfood Diet study lost a remarkable 7 pounds, including increased weight and muscle function. This dramatic impact on fat burning while encouraging muscles is one of the reasons why our Sirtfood diet is so popular with anyone who wants to get lean and healthy, including professional sportsmen and models who support this way of eating. In combination with fat burning, Sirtfoods also have the unique ability to satiate natural appetite, making them the ideal solution for a healthy weight and long-term sustainability. But considering it simply as a weight loss diet is a mistake. It's a diet that is as well-being a waistline. The nice 'side effects' of this way of eating are greater stamina, clearer skin, more alertness, and better sleep. The advantages are even more important, particularly in situations where metabolic disorders are reversed in the long term after a diet. These are their health improvements that studies show they are more powerful than prescription medicines to prevent chronic illnesses, with only a few benefits in diabetes, heart disease, and Alzheimer's. It is not surprising that it is well established that Sirtfoods are the leanest and healthiest in the world in cultures eating the most. The sirt foods have a range of health benefits in addition to weight loss. These health benefits should make it clear why you want these enriched food items. You know all the sirt foods and let's talk about their benefits.

It reduces cancer opportunities

Parsley is rich in vitamin C and flavonoid antioxidants, reducing oxidative stress in the body and raising the risk of certain cancers. A high intake of flavonoids in the diet, for example, can minimize the risk of colon cancer by up to 30%.

Buckwheat

Enhances the health of the heart

This seed-like grain helps reduce inflammation and lower LDL or "bad cholesterol" levels that are critical to heart health. Rutin, the primary nutrient that provides the main cardiovascular benefits, is a form of phytonutrient and antioxidant that helps to regulate blood pressure and reduce cholesterol.

Chile's Bird's View

It is famous for weight reduction. These play a crucial role in increasing the body's metabolism. As a result, the body temperature is increased. More calories are consumed in order to return the body to its original temperature, through the metabolic cycle. Increased metabolism is good and will allow the use of surplus fats contained in various parts of the body. As you may have noted, a rise in metabolism contributes to a sweat loss. Rapid metabolism, proper digestion, and waste disposal can reduce the risk of accumulation of fat in the body. Capsaicin is the chemical compound in bird chili that causes a sensation of burning. The effects of this compound can vary from person to person. However, many people experience a burning sensation of the mouth, throat, and stomach when ingested. The ingestion of bird's eye chili, therefore, increases metabolism and reduces body weight.

Decreases sugar in the blood

This pseudo-cereal in the glycemic index is very small in relation to other entire grains — that means that the contents of carbohydrates are gradually absorbed into the bloodstream and therefore ensure a constant supply of energy. This nutritious seed helps to regulate diabetes by preventing a sudden blood sugar spike and can enhance insulin resistance.

It is free of gluten and non-allergenic

Although it is similar to whole grains such as wheat and barley, it is naturally gluten-free, making it a better option for those with celiac disease or grain allergy.

Dietary Fiber Rich

For each cup of cooked groats, this food contains 6 grams of dietary fiber. Dietary fiber helps keep food moving through the digestive tract easily, which can make you eat longer – which can be an opportunity to lose weight if you want. It is also cancer-proof.

Healthy Vegetarian Protein Source

This food is not only rich in vitamins and minerals but also an excellent source of plant protein that can be digested. The diet includes up to 14 grams of protein per 100 grams of portion and 12 different amino acids for growth and muscle synthesis. The protein content of certain beans and legumes is not that high, but higher than most whole grains.

Walnuts

Walnuts contain significant amounts of antioxidants that keep the immune system healthy and prevent the occurrence of the disease. Walnuts are vacuum cleaners themselves because they sweep numerous bugs into the digestive system. The snack food is also ideal for heart health and weight loss as a declared superfood because of its nutrient content.

(Rich in fatty acids Omega-3)

The fatty acids omega-3 in walnuts are also healthy for the brain. Feeding high in omega-3 fatty acids makes the nervous system healthy and enhances performance. They are anti-cancer as well.

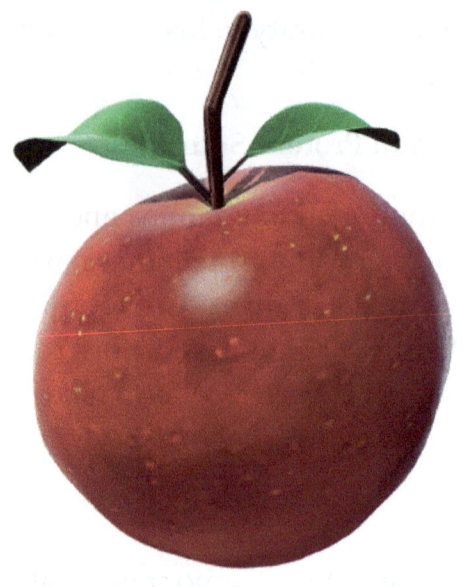

❖ 2.5 Common FAQs about the Sirtfood Diet

Is Sirtfoods for Children Suitable?

The Sirtfood diet is a powerful diet for weight loss and is not for children. However, it doesn't mean that children should miss more Sirtfoods for their remarkable health benefits in their general diets and help them receive a balanced, nutritious diet. Many of the recipes were prepared with families in mind, including kids' taste buds. Although most sirt foods are extremely healthy for children, green juices are not recommended since they are highly concentrated in fatty sirt foods. The caffeine present in coffee and green tea should also be protected from chilies. You can opt to keep it milder for kids.

What's the diet for Sirtfood?

"They recommend consuming different foods, which are nutritious foods, including, for example, broccoli, soy, and red wine. However, they also advocate limiting calories. They say, therefore, that they eat about 1000 calories per day for the first three days and then stick to about 1500 calories. You 're likely to lose weight if you take that amount of calories.

Is it safe?

"It is very difficult to determine whether it is safe or not, because no studies have looked at the diet in the long run. And if you limit yourself to 1000 calories per day, that's definitely not safe, especially if you're not in an environment that is medically supervised.

Why is it attractive?

"If I say to you that you can have your dark chocolate and your wine, I think your diet is more likely because you can eat things you like."

Do I need to practice during Phase 1?

A moderate and daily exercise increases the weight loss and health benefits of Phase 1 of the diet. It is suggested that you maintain your daily physical activity and exercise for the first seven days but stay in your usual comfort zone because too long or hard workouts will place too much stress on your body during this period. Listen to your body and instead let the Sirtfoods do the tough work.

Chapter 3: Getting Started with the Sirtfood Diet

The Sirtfood Diet promotes the consumption of fruit and vegetables that detoxify the body to prevent damage. Many people also love to eat chocolate and to drink red wine in their diet! Therefore, it is advisable to turn to sirtfood, a new dietary diet. The 23 top sirt foods form the basis of the Mediterranean and Japanese diets, with fewer people living with obesity and disease. In the Japanese, as in the Western world, five times as much food is consumed. It is crucial to find healthy eating and exercise routines that work, do not eliminate something you want, and do not allow you to practice with an estimated 650 million obese adults around the world during the week. That's what the Sirtfood diet is all about. The idea is that certain foods activate the paths of "skinny genes," often caused by fasting and exercise. Best of all, certain foods and beverages, including dark chocolate and red wine, contain the chemical materials known as polyphenols that activate the genes that imitate exercise and rapidity.

Exercise for the first few weeks Exercise for the first or two weeks of a diet would be sensitive to stop or reduce since your body sits at lower calories. Hear your body, and don't get tired or have less strength than normal. Please ensure you continue to focus on healthy living principles such as adequate daily fiber, protein, fruit, and vegetable concentrations. If you practice, it is necessary to eat protein, preferably one hour after practice. After exercise, the protein repairs your muscles and can help relieve sorrow. Several recipes contain a protein suitable for use after exercise, including sirt chili con carne, turmeric chicken, and kale salad. If you want something lighter and add protein powder to add interest, you should try a Sirt Blueberry Smoothie. The fitness you do is yours, but exercises at home will allow you to choose the type of exercise that's convenient and short.

Sirtfood is a great way to improve your eating habits, loss of weight, and healthy feelings. The first few weeks will challenge you but search for the best food to consume. Be kind to yourself in the first few weeks, when your body easily adapts and exercises if you decide. You can start as you usually do, or you can control fitness according to your diet adjustments if you are already a moderate or intense person. As with any changes in diet and exercise, the individual and how far you can go is all about.

❖ 3.1 Phases of Sirtfood Diet

The diet has two phases that are easy to follow:

PHASE 1: Seven days long. In the first three days, three green sirtfoods and one full sirtfood meal are to be provided – a total of 1,000 calories. From days 4 to 7, the calorie consumption will be increased to 1,500 with two green juices and two meals daily.

PHASE 2: This 14-day maintenance phase is designed to help you steadily lose weight. Three balanced sirtfood-rich meals, plus one green juice, are available every day. All steps can be replicated when you want to maximize the loss of fat.

- What's going on after phase two?
- And is this type of diet truly sustainable?

The idea of "sirtifying" meals is for those who have finished step 1 or 2 but want to proceed along the Sirtfood path. You must take your favorite dish and give it a sirtfood twist. Receptions include regular classics, including chicken curry, chili-con-carne, pizza, and pancakes.

The Sirtfood Diet is not intended as a one-off diet but as a way of life. You are advised to carry on consuming a diet rich in sirt food once you have completed the first three weeks and continue to drink your regular green juice. Many Sirtfood Diet recipe books with recipes for a lot more Sirtfood-rich main meals, as well as alternatives to green juice, and more tips for adopting the Sirtfood Diet, are available now. There are also some Sirtfood dessert recipes!

Phases 1 and 2 can be replicated if appropriate to boost our wellbeing or if things have gone a little off track.

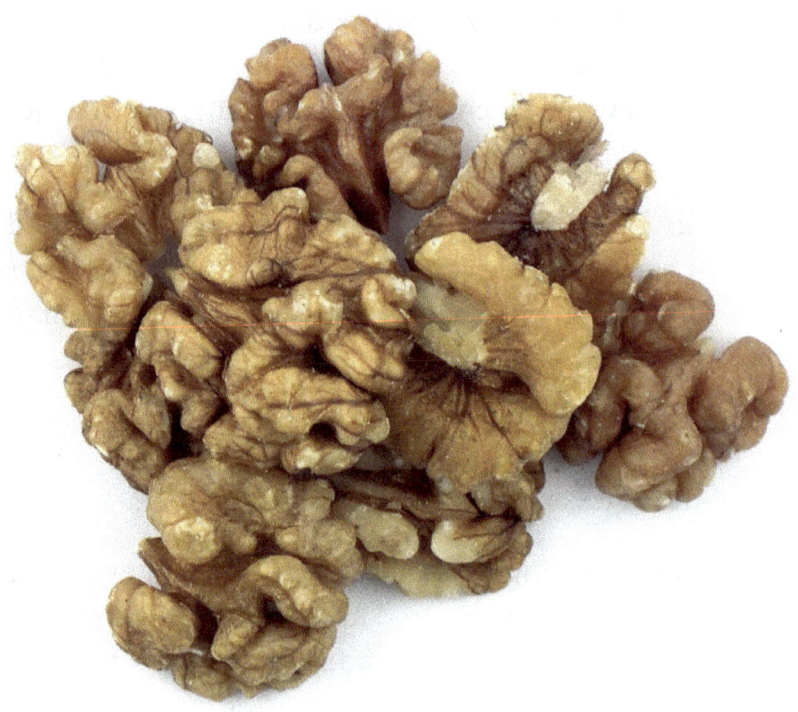

❖ 3.2 Shopping List of Sirtfood Diet Foods

Sounds like a snack taken straight from a science fiction film, "sirtfood" is a food high in Sirtuin activators, according to nutritionist Rob Hobson. Sirtuins are a type of protection against death or inflammation of the cells of our bodies, although research has also shown that they can help regulate your metabolism, increase your muscles, and burn fat – the new 'wonder food' label.

The headlines of the Sirtfood Diet are red wine and dark chocolate because both are high in sirtuin activators. Obviously, this isn't the entire picture, and the effects won't be felt by mainly Merlot and Green & Blacks (more pity). The Sirtfood Diet program focuses on increasing the intake of balanced meals. These are as follows:

- Red wine
- Citrus fruits
- Buckwheat
- Dark chocolate
- Medjool dates
- Parsley
- Walnuts
- Capers
- Green tea

- Blueberries
- Soy
- Turmeric
- Strawberries
- Olive oil
- Arugula
- Red onion
- Kale
- Apples

Interestingly enough, coffee is another highlight, which is welcome news when you're fed up with caffeine. Countries in which a wide variety of foods have already been eaten include Japan and Italy, which are currently among the healthiest countries in the world. There are 20 SIRT1-activating foods that can lose weight, reduce stubborn belly fat, and regain muscle mass in your diet.

You should also include chicken, beef and fish as sirtuin-activating foods are also present. However, these 20 should concentrate mainly on the plate.

Is there a diet schedule for Sirtfood?

Yes, there is.

Week 1:

- Drink three green sirtfoods a day

- Limit your daily intake to 1000 calories
- Eat a rich meal of sirtfood a day.

Week 2:

Up to 1500 calories a day

- Eat two meals full of sirtfoods a day.
- Drink two green sirtfood juices every day

There is no set strategy in the long run. It is about changing your lifestyle to make you feel better and more energetic with as many sirt foods as possible.

7-day diet schedule for sirtfood – phase 1 and phase 2

The Sirtfood diet continues with phase 1 in two phases – Stage 1 and Stage 2, every 3 and 4 days. Here is what to eat in phase 1 in the first stage.

Stage 1 (Day 1-3)

(1000 calories daily)

- 1/2 or 3/4 ounce 85% dark chocolate
- Three green juices a day
- Main options for meals
- One main meal a day
- Red Edamame, tomatoes, arugula and olive oil dressing buckwheat salad

- Arugula, chicken breast and walnuts dressed in strawberry and olive oil

- Walnut and olive oil salad with celery, kale, and capers

Step 2 (Day 4-Day 7)

(1500 calories daily)

- Two green juices a day
- Main options for meals
- Two primary meals a day
- Chicken cookie
- Soy chunks buckwheat noodles
- Muesli sirt
- Strawberry, roasting, and salad of walnut
- Salad of Waldorf
- Grilled red wine cod

Step 2: Week 2

You need to repeat what you did in the first week during the second week and maintain weight loss.

Following Phase 2

Here is what your diet schedule after 14 days of Sirtfood diet will look like:

- 3 healthy meals a day rich in sirtfood
- Sirtfood 1 or 2 snacks a day
- 1 Green sirtfood juice a day

❖ 3.3 Sirtfood Diet – 1 week of food plan

(Note: Please make your sample meal plan with 5 recipes per day (Breakfast-Snack 1-Lunch-Snack 2-Dinner) and place the meal plan in the next chapter).

The Sirtfood diet continues with phase 1 in two phases – Stage 1 and Stage 2, every 3 and 4 days. Here is what to eat in phase 1 in the first stage.

Stage 1 (Day 1-3)

(1000 calories daily)

- Three green juices a day

- 1/2 or 3/4 ounce 85% dark chocolate

- One main meal a day

- Main options for meals

- Walnut and olive oil salad with celery, kale, and capers

- Red Edamame, tomatoes, arugula and olive oil dressing buckwheat salad

- Arugula, chicken breast and walnuts dressed in strawberry and olive oil

Step 2 (Day 4-Day 7)

(1500 calories daily)

- Two green juices a day

- Main options for meals
- Two primary meals a day
- Chicken cookie
- Soy chunks buckwheat noodles
- Muesli sirt
- Strawberry, roasting, and salad of walnut
- Salad of Waldorf
- Grilled red wine cod

Chapter 4: Delicious Sirtfood Diet Recipes

❖ 4.1 Breakfast Recipes

This has been my meal for the past few weeks, and it's great. Indeed, I'm always on the SIRTfood way of eating – I love it, and I have plenty of strength and the weight I lost at first. And why change anything if it isn't right broken? If the spiciness of the pepper can't be treated, make sure you want it before throwing it into the pan, or you could be blown away.

1. SirtFood Scramble Mushroom Eggs

Ingredients:

- Two eggs
- 1 tsp turmeric field
- 1 tsp medium powder of curry
- 1 tsp of olive oil extra virgin
- 20 g broccoli, chopped roughly
- A handful of a champagne button, thinly sliced
- 1/2 chili of bird's eye, thinly sliced
- Fine chopped 5 g parsley
- * optional * Add a topper seed blend and taste a rooster sauce.

Directions

- Mix turmeric and curry powder and add a little water until a light paste is obtained.

- Steam the kale 2–3 minutes. Steam.

- In a pot, melt chili and champagne over medium heat for 2-3 minutes until browned and softened.

- Add the eggs and the spice paste to medium heat and cook the pear and cook for another minute over medium heat. Attach the parsley, blend, and serve well.

2. SALMON SALAD Baked with CREAMY MINT SIRTFOOD RECIPES

It's so easy to roast the Salmon in the oven.

Ready in 20 minutes

- 1 fillet of Salmon (130 g)
- 40 g young leaves of spinach
- 2 radishes, cut and sliced thinly
- 40 g blended leaves of salad
- 5 cm (50 g) slice of cucumber, cut into parts
- 1 small handful (10 g) parsley, chopped roughly
- 2 onions of spring, trimmed and sliced

For the dressing:

- Low-fat mayonnaise 1 tsp
- 1 tbsp. yogurt.
- 1 tbsp. vinegar of rice
- Salt and black pepper freshly ground
- 2 mint leaves, finely sliced.
- 1 Preheat the oven to 200 ° C (Fan / Gas 6 at 180 ° C).

1. Place the salmon fillet in a bakery and bake until only cooked for 16-18 minutes. Turn off the oven and set aside. The Salmon in the salad is just as hot or cold. If there is the skin on your Salmon, simply cook the skin and take the Salmon out of the skin after cooking with a piece of fish. When cooked, it should slide off easily.

2. Mix mayonnaise, yogurt, rice vinegar, mint leaves, and pepper and leave for at least 5 minutes in a small bowl.

3. Place salad leaves and spinach on a plate of service, and add the radishes, cucumber, spring onions and parsley on top. Float the cooked Salmon on the salad and drizzle over the dressing.

3. FRAGRANT ASIAN HOTPOT-SIRT FOOD RECIPES

(Calories 185)

Ready in 15 minutes

- 1 tsp of mashed tomato.
- Anise with 1 star, crushed (or 1/4 tsp anise)
- Small handful (10 g) cats, thinly sliced stalks
- 1/2 lime juice
- Small handful (10g) coriander, finely sliced stalks
- Chicken stock 500ml, new or made of 1 cube
- Split into tiny blooms 50 g broccoli
- 1/2 carrot, peeled and trimmed into matches.
- Fifty g beansprouts
- 100 g company tofu, cut.
- 100 g small tiger crevices
- 50 g rice noodles, cooked as instructed in the packet
- 20 g sushi ginger, split
- 50 g water chestnuts cooked, drained
- Good quality miso paste 1 tbsp.

Stir in the large pot and simmer for 10 minutes with the tomato purée, star anise, pelvis stalks, coriander stalks, lime juice, and chicken stock. Add carrot, broccoli, creeping plates, tofu, noodles, and water chestnuts and cook until the creeps are finished. Stir the sushi ginger and miso paste out of the heat. Serve with parsley and coriander leaves sprinkled.

4. Blackcurrant Compote-Sirtfood Recipes Apple Pancakes

(Calories 337)

These pancakes are healthy but decadent—a great lazy treat in the morning. Ready in twenty minutes.

- 75 g oats porridge
- 1 tsp baking powder
- 125 g plain flour
- Pinch of Salt
- 2 tbsp. sugar caster
- 2 peeled apples, cored and chopped into small pieces
- 2 white eggs
- Half-skimmed milk 300 ml
- Light olive oil 2 tsp

1- Render the compote first. In a small pan, place the blackcurrants, sugar, and tea. Bring to a frying pan and cook for 10-15 minutes.

2- In a large bowl, put oats, meal, bakery powder, caster sugar, and salt and mix well. Attach the apple and whisk a little at a time into the milk until the mixture is smooth. Whisk the egg whites into steep peaks and fold them into the batter. Transfer to a jug the batter.

3- Boil 1/2 tsp oil in a non-stick dish over medium-high heat and pour in about a quarter of the butter. Cook until golden brown on both sides. Repeat to make four pancakes.

4- Serve the blackcurrant compote over the pancakes.

5. SIRT MUESLI-SIRT FOOD RECIPE

Ingredients:

- 20 g flakes of buckwheat
- 15 g flakes of cocoa or desiccated cocoa
- 10 g puffs of buckwheat
- 40 g Dates of Medjool, pitted and chopped
- 10 g nibs of cocoa
- Hulled and chopped 100 g of strawberries
- Walnuts 15 g, cut 15 g
- 100 g Greek plain yogurt (or another vegan, such as soy or coconut yogurt)

Directions:

Combine all of the above ingredients, adding yogurt and strawberries right before serving, if it is done in bulk.

❖ 4.2 Sirtfood Diet Juices and Drinks

1. KALE AND BLACKCURRANT SMOOTHIE-SIRT FOOD RECIPES

(Calories 86)

Ready in 3 minutes

- 2 tsp honey
- 10 baby kale leaves, removed stalks
- 1 cup of new green tea
- 40 g blackcurrants, stalks and washed away
- 1 mature banana
- 6 cubes of ice

Mix the sweetheart in the moist green tea until it dissolves. Whisk all ingredients smoothly in a blender. Serve immediately. Serve immediately.

❖ 4.3 Lunch Recipes

This dish explodes with so many delicious flavors that you can forget that you eat it. Only one FYI on chili – I just love spicy food, so I use the whole Thai chili, even the grains, but first, I would suggest extracting the seeds to see how much heat they can withstand.

1. Spiced cauliflower chicken couscous

Ingredients:

- 150 g chopped or processed cauliflower (1 cup)
- 10 g flat parsley leafed
- 100 g (1 breast) 100 g chicken
- Two tsp soil Turmeric
- Fine diced carrots of 40 g (1/4 cup)
- 1 garlic clove, thinly diced
- Good diced 40 g red onions (1/4 cup)
- 1 tsp of fresh ginger finely chopped
- 1 chili bird 's head, cut (Thai chili)
- 2 EVOO Tbsp.
- 1/2 lemon juice
- Tomatoes with 30 g sun-dried (less than 1/4 cup)
- 1 Tbsp. capers

Directions

- In the food processor or roughly chop couscous, set aside.

- Heat 1 tbsp. of EVOO over medium heat in pan-add chili, ginger, and garlic and sprinkle until smooth but not coloring.

- Remove turmeric, cauliflower, and carrots and cook for a few minutes.

- Remove from heat and mix with tomatoes in a bowl and reserve parsley.

- Use the other 1 tbsp. of oil on each side and cook the chicken for about 5 to 6 minutes, then add lemon juice, capers, and 1 tbsp. of water to the pot once cooked (165 F).

- Combine rice, "sauce" and couscous, and serve together.

2. HONEY LIME TOURMERY DRESSING-SIRTFOOD RECIPES & KALE SALAD

Time to schedule: Twenty minutes

Time to cook: 10 minutes

Overall period: Thirty minutes

Notes: Dress the salad in advance 10 minutes before serving. Beef small, chopped prawns or fish may replace chicken. Vegetarians can use chopped or cooked quinoa mushrooms.

Service: 2

Ingredients:

For the poultry

- 1 tea cubicle ghee or 1 tbsp. cocoon oil
- 250-300 g / 9 ounces. Chicken thin or chicken thighs diced
- 1/2 brown onion small, diced.
- 1 big clove of garlic, fine diced.
- 1 thirty cubic metal zest
- 1 turmeric teaspoon powder
- 1/2 lime juice
- 1/2 teaspoon of salt + potato.

For the salad

- 6 stalks of broccoli or 2 cups of broccoli.
- 3 big kale leaves, cut and removed stems
- 2 potted cucumber seeds (pipits)
- handful of fresh leaves of chopped coriander
- 1/2 prosecutor
- handful of fresh, chopped piglet leaves

For the dressing

- 3 cubicle lime juice

- 3 extra virgin olive oil tablespoons (I used 1 tablespoon of avocado oil and 1 tablespoon of EVO).

- 1 small, thinly diced or rubbed a garlic clove

- 1 teaspoon raw sweetheart

- 1/2 tea cubicle salt and pepper

- 1/2 full-grain teaspoon of Dijon mustard

Instructions

1. Heat ghee or cocoa oil over medium-high heat in a small frying pan. Add the onion and sauté at medium heat for 4-5 minutes, until golden. Add chicken thin and garlic and run for 2-3 minutes at medium-high heat.

2. Add the turmeric, lime zest, limestone juice, salt, and pepper and cook for another 3-4 minutes, mixing frequently. Set aside the cooked thinness.

3. Hold a small cup of water to boil while the chicken is cooking. Add breadcrumbs and cook for 2 minutes. Rinse and cut into three to four pieces, each under cold water.

4. Attach the potato seeds to the chicken frying pan and toast for 2 minutes over medium heat, regularly mixing to avoid burning. Season with a small amount of salt. Set aside. Set aside. Raw pumpkin seeds are perfect for use as well.

5. Put the chopped kale in a bowl of salad and pour over the dressing. Toss and rub the kale with the dressing with your fingertips. The kale softens like citrus juice for fish or beef carpaccio – it 'cooks' it slightly.

6. Then toss the cooked chicken, broccoli, fresh herbs, seeds, and slices of avocados.

3. CHICKEN KALE & MISO Dressing-SIRTFOOD RECIPES BUCKWHEAT NOODLES

Prep time: 15 minutes

Cook time: 15 minutes

Total time: 30 minutes

Service: 2

Ingredients:

For the nudges

- 2-3 pounds of kale leaves (roughly cut from the stem)
- 3-4 mushroom shiitake
- Buckwheat noodles 150 g / 5 oz. (100% buckwheat, no wheat)
- 1 brown onion, thinly diced
- 1 tablespoon of ghee or cocoa oil
- 1 small, sliced, or diced chicken breast.
- 2 big, thinly diced garlic cloves.
- 1 long, thinly sliced red chili (seeds inside or out, depending on how hot you like it).

- Tamari sauce (gluten-free soy sauce) for 2-3 tablespoons.

For the miso dressing:

- 1 1/2 cubic meter new biological miso
- 1 extra virgin olive oil spoon
- 1 cucharco Tamari sauce
- Sesame oil (optional) 1 teaspoon.
- One tablespoon of citrus fruit or lime juice

Instructions:

1. Take to boil a medium bowl of water. Add the kale and cook until slightly wilted for 1 minute. Remove and reserve the water but bring it back to the boil. Add the soba noodles and cook (normally about 5 minutes) according to package instructions. Rinse and set aside under cold water.

2. Alternatively, cook the shiitake mushrooms for 2-3 minutes in small ghee or coconut oil (about a teaspoon), and brown slightly on each side. Sprinkle the salt of the sea and reserve.

3. Steam more coconut oil or ghee in the same frying pot over medium-high heat. Pour in the onion and chili and add the chicken pieces for 2-3 minutes. Cook over medium heat for 5 minutes, stirring a few times, adding garlic, tamari sauce, and a small bubble of water. Cook for another 2-3 minutes, stir until the chicken is cooked.

4. Finally, add the noodles of kale and soba and toss the chicken to warm up.

5. At the end of cooking, mix the miso and drizzle over the noodles, thus keeping all the beneficial probiotics alive and active in the miso.

4. SIRT FOOD RECIPES ASIA KING STIR-FRY with BUCKWHEAT NOODLES

Serving 1

Ingredients:

- 150 g of raw king prawns shelled, deveined
- Extra virgin olive oil 2 tsp
- 2 tsp tamari (if you don't avoid gluten you can use soy sauce)
- 75 g soba (noodles of buckwheat)
- 1 chili bird's eye, finely chopped
- 1 clove of garlic, finely chopped
- 1 tsp of fresh ginger finely chopped
- Celery 40 g, cut and trimmed
- Sliced 20 g red onions 20 g
- 75 g green beans, split
- Chicken stock 100ml

- 5 g lovage or celery leaves

- 50 g broccoli, chopped roughly

Heat a frying pan high heat and bake the creams for 2-3 minutes in 1 teaspoon tamari and 1 teaspoon of oil. Transfer the creeping things to a plate. Wipe the pan out with paper from the kitchen, as you will use it again.

Cook the noodles for 5–8 minutes in boiling water or as directed. Drain and reserve. In the meantime, fry the garlic, chili, and ginger, red onion, celery, boar, and chalk in the remaining oil for 2 to 3 minutes over medium-high heat. Add stock and bring to a boil. Simmer until the vegetables are cooked and crooked for a minute or two. Add the crew, noodles, and lavage/celery leaves to the pot, then take them back to boil and serve.

❖ 4.4 Sirtfood Diet Salad Recipes

1. BUCKWHEAT PASTA SALAD-SIRT FOOD RECIPE

Serving 1

- Pasta buckwheat 50 g (cooked as instructed by the packet)
- A small handful of leaves of basil
- A small handful of rockets
- 10 olive trees
- 8 tomatoes or cherry, halved
- Pine nuts 20 g
- Extra virgin olive oil 1 tbsp.

Combine all ingredients carefully except pine nuts and arrange them in a dish or cup, then scatter the pine nuts over the rim.

2. SKEWERS SIRT FOOD RECIPE: GREEK SALAD

Ready in 10 minutes

- 2 wooden skewers, 30 minutes before use, immersed in water
- Eight tomatoes of cherry
- 1 yellow pepper, eight squares split
- Eight big black olives

- 1/2 red onions, halved and 8 pieces separated.
- Feta 100 g, divided into eight cubes
- 100 g (10 cm) of cucumber, sliced into four slices and halved.

For the dressing:

- Extra virgin olive oil 1 tbsp.
- 1 tsp of vinegar balsamic
- 1/2 lemon juice
- 1/2 garlic clove, skinned and crushed
- Few oregano leaves, finely chopped
- Generous salt and fresh ground black pepper seasoning
- Few basil leaves, fine chopped (or 1/2 tsp of dried mixed herbs for the substitution of basil and oregano)
- 1 Thread the salad ingredients into each skewer: olives, tomatoes, yellow pepper, red onions, cucumber, basil, olives, red oak, cucumber, feta.

In a small bowl, put all the dressing ingredients and blend thoroughly together. Put the skewers over.

3. SESAME SALAD-Sirt food Recipe

304 cals

Serve: 2

Ready in 12 minutes

A delicious and extraordinary salad.

- 1 sesame tbsp. seeds
- 100 g baby kale, chopped roughly
- 1 cucumber, peeled, halfway through, desired with a teaspoon and sliced
- 60 g bag choi, shredded very finely
- A small handful (20 g) of chopped parsley
- 1/2 red onions, very sliced
- 150 g of chicken fried, shredded

For the dressing:

- Extra virgin olive oil 1 tbsp
- 1 lime juice
- 1 tsp of his own oil
- Sauce of 2 tsp soy
- 1 tsp transparent darling

Instructions:

1- Toast seeds of sesame for 2 minutes, slightly browned and fragrant, in a dry frying pan. Transfer to a cooling plate.

2- Blend olive oil, sesame oil, lime juice, honey, and soy sauce together in a small bowl for dressing.

3- Put in a wide bowl the cucumber, kale, pak choi, red onion, and parsley, and combine well. Put the dressing over and blend again.

4- Spread the salad between two plates and top with chicken shredded. Just before eating, brush over the sesame seeds.

6. Strong Salad-Sirtfood Salmon Sirt Recipes

Serves: 1

Ingredients:

- Rocket 50 g
- 100 g smoked salmon slices (lenses, cooked chicken breast or tinned tuna may also be used)
- 50 g leaves of chicory
- Avocado 80 g, with peeling, stoning and sliced
- Sliced 20 g red onion
- Sliced 40 g celery
- Walnuts 15 g, cut 15 g
- 1 big date of Medjool, pitted and cut
- 1 tbsp. of cables
- Extra virgin olive oil 1 tbsp.
- 1Parsley 10 g, chopped
- /4 lemon juice
- 10 g lifting or celery leaves, cut

Process:

Place the salad leaves on a large plate. Combine all the other ingredients and serve on top of the leaves.

❖ 4.5 Dinner Recipes

1. LAMB SIRT FOOD DATE AND BUTTERNUT SQUASH

Time to schedule: Fifteen minutes

Time to cook: 1 hour and 15 minutes

Overall period: 1 hour and 30 minutes

Service: 4

Unbelievable Moroccan warming spices make this safe day perfect for snowy autumn and winter nights. Serve with buckwheat for an additional boost in safety!

Ingredients:

- 2 cup harks of olive oil.
- Ginger 2 cm, grated
- 3 cloves of garlic grated or crushed
- Sliced 1 red onion
- 1 tablespoon flakes of chili (or taste)
- 1 piece of cinnamon
- 2 tea cubes of cumin seeds
- 2 teaspoons of turmeric ground
- 1/2 tea cubicle salt

- 800 g fillet lamb back, cut into 2 cm chunks
- Dates of 100 g Medjool, pitted and chopped
- 500 g squash butternut, cut into 1 cm cubes
- 400 g of tomatoes diced, plus half a bowl of water
- Drained 400 g canned chickpeas
- Buckwheat, couscous or rice to serve
- new coriander 2 tablespoons (plus extra garnish)

Process:

1. Preheat your 140C oven.

2. Drizzle around 2 olive oil tablespoons into a large ovenproof casserole dish or cast-iron casserole. Slice onion and cook for about 5 minutes in a gentle heat, until the onions are softened, but not browned.

3. Add the garlic, chili, cumin, cinnamon, and turmeric grated. Stir well and cook with the lid for another 1 minute. If it gets too dry, add a splash of water.

4. Next, add pieces of lamb. Add salt, chopped dates, and tomatoes, plus about half a can of water (100-200ml) to cover the meat in the ointment and spices.

5. Take the tagine to the boil and put the lid on and put 1 hour and 15 minutes in your pre-heated oven.

6. Add chopped butternut squash and dried chickpeas thirty minutes before the end of the cooking time. Remove all

together, put the lid back on, and return to the oven for the last 30 minutes.

7. Once the tagine is finished, remove the coriander from the oven and cook it. Serve with buckwheat, couscous, rice, or basmati.

Remarks:

If you don't have an ovenproof casserole pot or cast-iron casserole, cook the tagine simply in a regular casserole until it's in the oven and transfer it into a regular casserole pot before putting it in the oven. Apply an additional five minutes to prepare, so that the casserole dish has more time to heat up.

2. PRAWN ARRABBIATA-SIRT FOOD RECIPE

Serving 1

Time for preparation: 35 – forty minutes

Prep time: 20 – 30 min.

Ingredients:

- 65 g Pasta Buckwheat

- 125-150 g Raw or cooked crevasses (ideally king crevasses)

- Extra virgin olive oil 1 tbsp.

For sauce of arrabbiata

- 40 g Red onion, thinly sliced

- 30 g Celery, thinly cut.
- 1 clove of garlic, finely chopped
- 1 tsp Dried herbs 1 tsp
- 1 Bird's eye chili, chopped finely
- Extra virgin olive oil 1 tsp
- 400 g Tinned tomatoes chopped
- White wine 2 tbsp. (optional)
- 1 tbsp. Petroleum chopped

Process:

1. Cook onion, garlic, celery, chili, and herbs in the oil for 1-2 minutes, at medium-low heat. Turn the heat to average, add the wine and cook for 1 minute. Attach the tomatoes and let the sauce cook for 20-30 minutes on medium-low heat until it has a good rich consistency. When the sauce gets too thick, just add a little water.

2. Grab a pot of water to a boil during cooking and prepare pasta in compliance with package instructions. Drain, add the olive oil and keep it in the pot until appropriate when cooked to your taste.

3. When you have simple crevices, apply it to the sauce and cook 3-4 minutes longer until it is pink and opaque, apply the parsley and serve. When cooked creams are used, add the parsley to them, bring the sauce to the boil and serve.

4. In the sauce, mix thoroughly, but gently, and serve the cooked pasta.

3. Fried POTATOES AS Fried STEW-SIRT FOOD RECIPE

Time to schedule: 10 minutes

Time to cook: One hour

Serving: 4-6

The Spicy Chickpea Stew is unbelievably delicious and a great top for baked potatoes and just vegetarian, vegan, gluten-free, and leather-free. Especially Mexican Mole meets North African Tagine. And the chocolate is there.

Ingredients:

- 4-6 fried, baked potatoes all over
- 2 red onions, smoothly cut
- 2 cu harks of olive oil.
- Ginger 2 cm, grated
- 4 garlic cloves, rubbed or crushed
- Chili flakes (just as hot as you like) 1/2 to 2 teaspoons
- 2 turmeric teaspoons
- 2 cubic metal cumin seeds
- Hot splash

- 2 unsweetened teaspoons of cocoa powder (or chocolate)

- Tomatoes 2 x 400 g tins

- 2 yellow peppers (or whatever color you like!), chopped in pieces of bitesize

- 2 x 400 g of tins of chickpeas (or, if you prefer, kidney beans) including chickpea water NOT DRAIN!!

- 2 extra tablespoons of parsley for garnish

- Side salad (facultative)

- Salt and pepper (optional) to taste

Process:

1. Preheat the oven to 200C before all of your ingredients can be packed.

2. When it's hot enough, put in the oven and cook your bakery potatoes for 1 hour or until you're done as you like them.

3. When the potatoes have been in the oven, put the olives oil and chopped red onion in a wide cup and boil carefully, lid on them for 5 minutes, until the onions are mild but not brown.

4. Pull off the cover and then apply the garlic, ginger, cumin, and chili. Cook at low heat for another minute, add turmeric and a very small sprinkle of water and cook for another minute so that the pot is not too hot.

5. Add tomatoes, powdered cocoa (or cacao), chickpeas (including water chickpea), and pepper yellow. Bring to boil, then cook for 45 minutes at low heat until the sauce is thick and smooth (but don't let it burn!). The stew should be made approximately at the same time as the potatoes.

6. Finally, add 2 tablespoons of parsley, salt, and pepper if you like to and serve the stew with a simple side salad on top of baked potatoes.

3- Cook onion for 5-7 minutes in 1 teaspoon of oil over medium heat until soft and nicely caramelized. Keep dry. Keep warm. Steam the kale 2-3 minutes and drain. In 1/2 teaspoon of oil fry the garlic for 1 minute gently until soft, but not colored. Add the kale and fry until tender for another 1-2 minutes. Keep dry. Keep warm.

4- Heat the ovenproof frying pot to smoke and overheat. Coat the meat in 1/2 teaspoon of oil and fry it in the hot pot over medium-high heat, as your meat is done. If you like the medium, sew meat and then move it into a 220 oC / gas 7 stove and then finish the cooking at the prescribed times.

5- Take the meat out of the bowl and set aside for rest. Attach the wine to the hot pot to absorb any traces of meat — bubble to halve the wine until it has a syrupy and concentrated flavor.

6- Add the bowl and the tomato paste to the steak pan and then bring to a boil, then add the paste from corn flour to thicken the sauce and add until you have a perfect consistency. Attach the rusty steaks in some juice and eat the roasted potatoes, broccoli, onion rings, and red sauce of the wine.

❖ 4.6 Sirtfood Diet Dessert Recipes

1. CHOCOLATE CUPCAKES WITH MATCHA ICING-SIRT FOOD RECIPES

234 calories

Serves: 12

Ready in 35 minutes

- 150 g self-raising meal
- Cocoa 60 g
- 200 grams of caster sugar
- Salt 1/2 tsp.
- 120 ml of dairy
- 1/2 tsp coffee with a perfect espresso, decaf if desired
- Extract 1/2 tsp of vanilla
- 1 egg
- Vegetable oil 50ml
- Boiling water of 120 ml

For the refrigeration:

- At room temperature 50 g butter
- Drop 1 tbsp. matcha green tea

- 50 g sugar icing
- Soft cream from 50 g
- 1/2 tsp of bean paste

Process:

1- Preheat the oven to the fan of 180C/160C. Line the paper or silicone cupcake tin. Line the cupcake tin.

2- In a wide bowl, put flour, sugar, cacao, salt, and espresso powder and thoroughly combine.

3- Add to the dry ingredients milk, vanilla extract, vegetable oil and egg, and use an electric mixer to beat well. Put the boiling water carefully slowly and bathe at low speed until completely combined. Use high speed to beat the butter for another minute. The batter is much more liquid than a normal mixture of cake. Have confidence, and it's going to taste amazing!

4- Spoon the batter between the cake cases equally. No more than 3/4 complete should be used for each cake event. Bake 15-18 minutes in the oven before the mixture bounces back. Remove from the oven and cool until freezing absolutely.

5- Mix together the butter and the icing sugar until light and smooth to create the icing. Remove the matcha and vanilla powder and blend again. Then add the cream cheese and beat until it is smooth. Pipe or scatter across the cakes.

2. Jelly-Sirtfood Raspberry and Blackcurrant Recipes

Calories: 76

Serving: 2

Available in 15 minutes + time setting

Making a jelly beforehand is an excellent way of preparing the fruit to be ready first in the morning.

- A hundred grams of raspberry washed
- 100 g of cassava, washed and cut stalks
- 2 gelatin leaves
- Water 300ml
- 2 tbsp. sugar granulated

Process:

1- Place the raspberries in two dishes/glasses/molds. In a bowl of cold water, place gelatin leaves to soften.

2- Put the blackcurrants in a small pot with 100ml water and sugar and bring to a boil. Simmer vigorously and remove from heat for 5 minutes. Leave 2 minutes to stand.

3- Suck the excess water out of the gelatin leaves and return it to the cup. Remove until dissolved, then add the rest of the bath. In the prepared dishes, add the liquid and cool it to place. The jellies should be ready for approximately 3-4 hours.

Conclusion

This book would be all you need to start your weight loss journey if you are sick of your continuous cycle of unhealthy and unsatisfying diet. This book packs in it the ultimate advice to start with your Sirtfood diet. The book not only addresses questions such as what is a Sirtfood diet but will also explain and show you how you can start following it for your own benefit. Sirtfood is really a superior diet to not only vegan but also to other mainstream diets such as the carnivore diet devised by John Baker. The main purpose of Sirtfood diet revolves around activating a very specialized protein in the body known as the Sirtuins, the sirtuins are the proteins whose main purpose is to stop cells from dying out under stress and thus contributes to less ageing as well as higher metabolism. The purpose of writing this book is to show people how great of a diet it is and how it could benefit you by not only improving your appearances but also by improving your state of mind by making it clearer, as it has benefitted many other people including many celebrities such as the pop singer Adele. The book will dive into the history of Sirtfood diet so as to see what led to its origination and to properly understand how it works. To get you started out on this amazing journey of Sirtfood diet the book also includes a wide range of delicious recipes that you can try out. These recipes are so tasty that don't even let you feel that you are on any kind of diet. Such is the amazingness of a Sirtfood diet..

www.ingramcontent.com/pod-product-compliance
Lightning Source LLC
Chambersburg PA
CBHW070032040426
42333CB00040B/1573